Healthy Eating for Children

The Power of Organic Food

Natural Health Series

Dueep J. Singh

Mendon Cottage Books

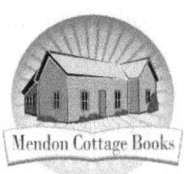

JD-Biz Publishing

All Rights Reserved.

Disclaimer

The information is this book is provided for informational purposes only. It is not intended to be used and medical advice or a substitute for proper medical treatment by a qualified health care provider. The information is believed to be accurate as presented based on research by the author.

The contents have not been evaluated by the U.S. Food and Drug Administration or any other Government or Health Organization and the contents in this book are not to be used to treat cure or prevent disease.

The author or publisher is not responsible for the use or safety of any diet, procedure or treatment mentioned in this book. The author or publisher is not responsible for errors or omissions that may exist.

Warning

The Book is for informational purposes only and before taking on any diet, treatment or medical procedure, it is recommended to consult with your primary health care provider.

Check out some of the other Healthy Gardening Series books at Amazon.com

Gardening Series on Amazon

Check out some of the other Health Learning Series books at Amazon.com

Health Learning Series on Amazon

Table of Contents

Introduction 4

Fussy Kids 7

Introducing Organic Eating 9

Organic Foods 12

Pesticides in Food 16

Organic Junk Foods… 18

Taste and Nutritional Benefits 21

Cost Factor 25

No Chemicals 27

Healthy Eating Outdoors 31

Different Food Textures 33

Safety Tips While Eating Outdoors 35

Conclusion 38

Author Bio 39

Publisher 49

Introduction

You may have noticed that a large number of parents around you are quite worried about the quality of the food eaten by their children. It is possible that you are of that number.

A sensible parent knows that establishing the foundation of excellent and long-lasting health throughout his child's lifetime needs to be set during babyhood itself. The main priority here is giving them excellent nourishing, high quality and good food.

So it doesn't matter whether you are a parent or a guardian, a child minder or a teacher – the tips and techniques for healthy eating, especially encouraging the children under your responsibility to learn to appreciate organic food – is going to depend on you.

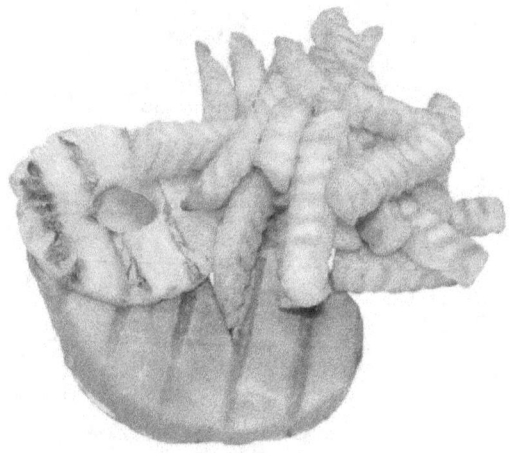

This comes under the category of healthy eating, if the potato chips , and meat is barbecued/roasted and not fried.

Eating nutritious food, especially when it is healthy is going to give your child the basis of good health, a strong physical and mental presence and a long-term immunity against illnesses and diseases.

One of the most important health messages which are aimed at children's health is being neglected in the 21st century. In ancient times, children were encouraged to go out in the gardens, and pick fresh fruit and vegetables as often as they could, and eat them. In fact, in ancient times, when there was no junk food around, vegetables and fruit were given to children in such abundance that you could count about five helpings in a day fed to them.

And because they were as hungry as little wolves, having done plenty of exercise and physical labor, in the fields and outdoors, they did not get a chance of saying "I do not like this. I am not going to eat this. Where are my hamburgers? Where are my French fries? Where is my sugar-based fizzy pop? Vegetables –blecch!"

Any child throwing such a tantrum on the dinner table was immediately disciplined and sent off to bed hungry. That taught him that meals needed to be eaten without further Ado or tantrums, because the alternative was no meals.

Unfortunately, in the 21st century, we allow children to eat whatever they want, because we could not be bothered about feeding them nutritious diets. The advertising in the food brand market is focused on children as future clients. That is why unhealthy foods, especially junk foods are so much in demand today.

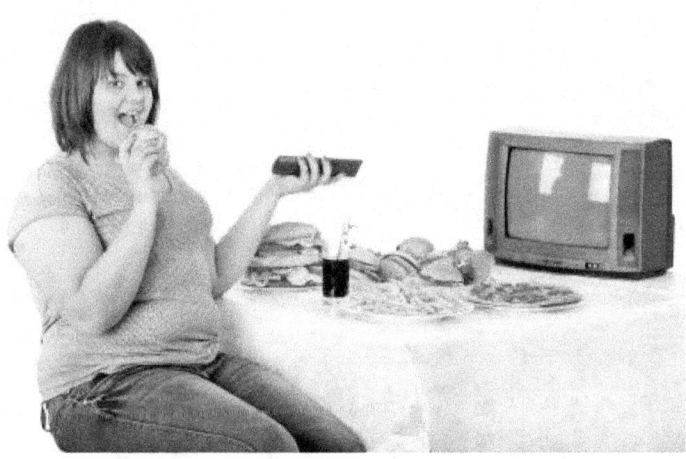

These unhealthy eating habits started in childhood.

As the hectic lifestyles of parents allow them less and less time for cooking, and junk foods beckon attractively and the consumers from supermarket shelves, is it a surprise that children's health is suffering accordingly? Believe it or not, children ate healthier in the 1950s, because mothers knew about proper nourishing diets. They also took the time to cook healthy, nourishing meals for their children. Not many mothers do that today, when all they have to do is open up a soup can, and heat it in the microwave.

So if you are a parent and are wondering how to encourage your children to eat vegetables, what is an organic diet, what to do about a child who fusses about his meals, and how can you feed your child in a healthy manner, this is the book for you.

Fussy Kids

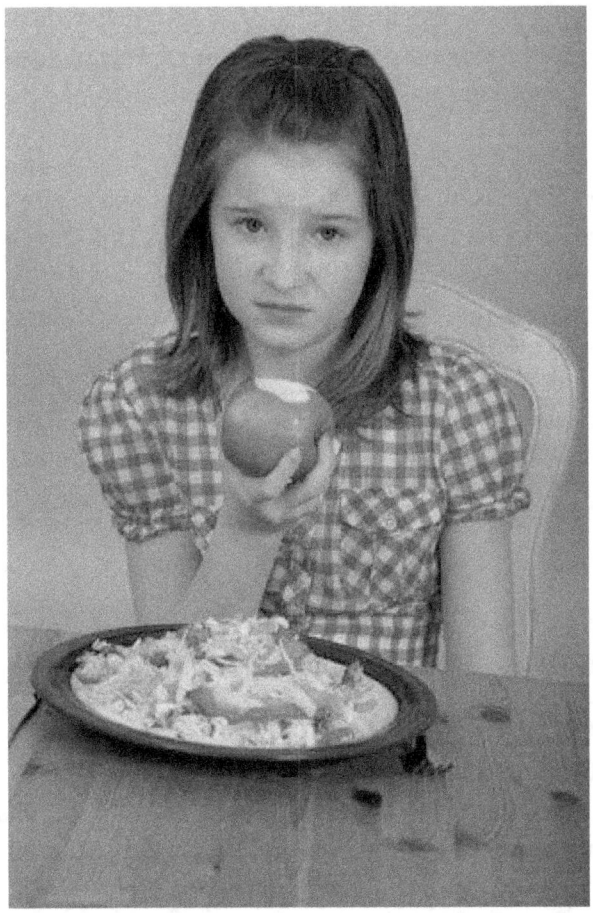

Boring, boring... Not at all tasty.

Many parents have lost the knack of disciplining their children, especially when it is time to eat. That is because the children have been allowed to gain the upper hand, in dictating what they want to eat, and the parents take the line of least resistance in order to keep peace in the family.

That is why, children who enjoy pushing the buttons of the parents, in order to see how far they can go before they are disciplined start making fusses about eating.

I remember once as a child, I decided to do the same thing. There was custard pudding on the table, and I made a face. Being a rather spoiled brat, I wanted my parents to cajole me into eating the pudding, and then I would relent. Instead, my father quietly picked up my bowl of delicious, mouthwatering custard pudding, and placed it in front of my younger brother, who finished it in the twinkling of an eye.

Then my father said, "Okay, so you do not like custard pudding? You need not eat it, ever again. Your brother is going to have your share, from now on. This goes for everything you do not eat. The food is delicious and tasty. If you do not eat it, you do not get it. Stay hungry. You are now excused from the table and can go to your room."

I looked at him open- mouthed. This was retribution with a vengeance. I could not even go back on my decision, and say, "no, no, I liked, I loved custard pudding."

Since that day I ate what was put in front of me quietly and without any fuss.

So the moral of the story is if the child is taught to fuss when he is a baby, and the parents do not discipline him in the beginning itself, he is going to grow up to be a fussy eater.

The habit of allowing children to sneak snacks and other things to eat, in between meals is another way in which you can encourage bad eating habits. We were definitely not allowed to have snacks and biscuits in our bedrooms. If we felt hungry – being normal, active children – after an hour of playing outdoors, we came in and we were fed a glassful of milk and some fruit. That was enough to tide us over until the next mealtime.

Remember that it is not very complicated to inculcate good eating habits in your children. However, it is going to need a degree of discipline, time, inclination, and also common sense, determination and consistency. Do not allow pester power to undermine your status of alpha dog in the family.

This is where healthy eating, especially organic food, eating comes in.

Introducing Organic Eating

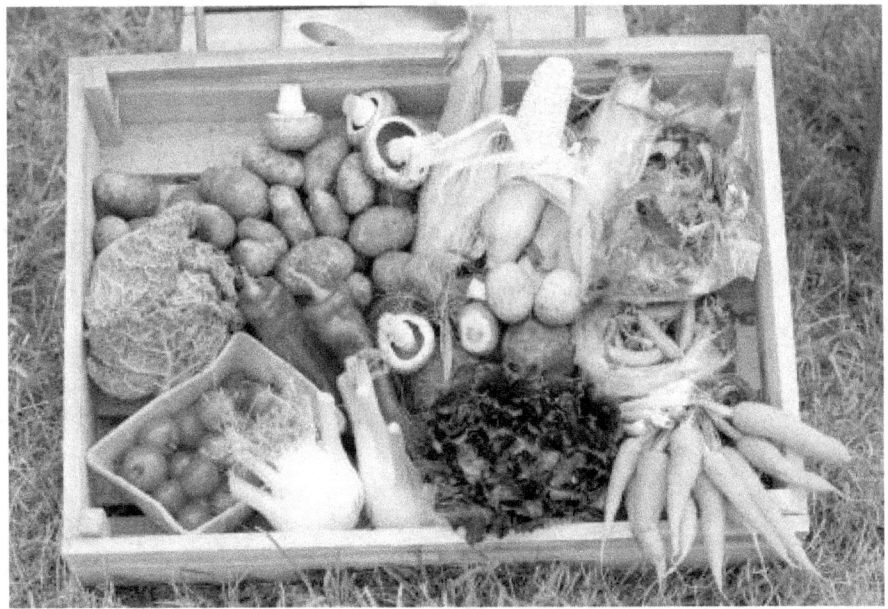

Having children is a great responsibility. It also means that you need to change your lifestyle in such a manner, that your children have access to your time. The basic foundation of a healthy childhood is going to be based on attending to your children's nutritional needs.

This is going to include cooking healthy meals, and feeding fresh food to your family. Obviously, the earlier you can help your children to establish good eating habits, the more easily, they are going to accept the fact that whatever is put on the table is tasty, delicious and healthy.

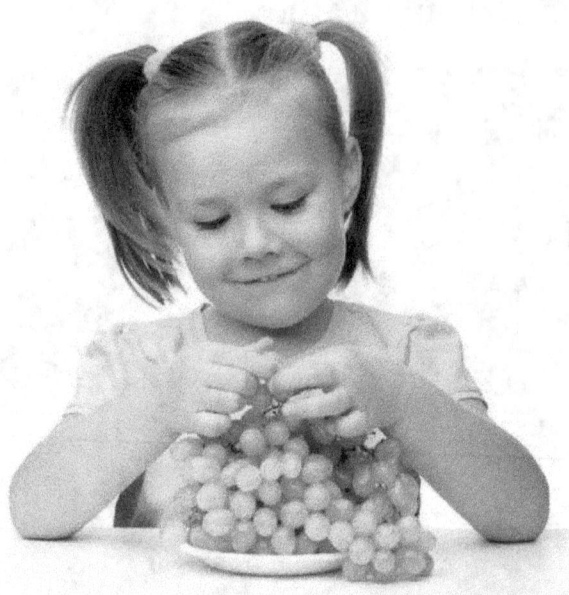

Do not ever say "Eat this, this is good for you." Instead, if the children see you eating a particular food, without any fuss, they are going to follow you.

Children are great imitators. Also, they want to eat whatever their parents eat. So if you are subsisting on junk food, it is a given that they are also going to start eating junk food as a matter of course. On the other hand, if parents are sensible enough to eat healthy, nutritional food as a part of their daily diets, it is a given that their children are also going to do the same thing.

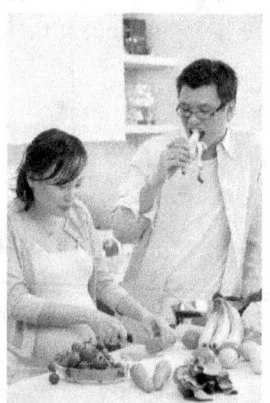

Healthy eating lifestyles followed by responsible parents means healthy new generations in the future.

Children can easily influenced or be waylaid by any number of health demolishing habits, including fast food, soft drink advertisements, heavily advertised food for kids, and also sedentary lifestyles.

So once you recognize the fact that you need to change the eating habits of your children, as well as of your family, there will soon come a time when your children will begin to appreciate and savor good food. They may also enjoy learning how to prepare healthy meals, in which organic foods are going to play a major part.

More than USD300 million are spent in the USA alone on organic food, and there is going to be a significant rise in this amount as more and more people start deciding to eat organic.

So how come "Developed" countries are spending so much money on "organic" food? And what is this?

Organic Foods

Organic foods mean –

No use of artificial fertilizer and artificial pesticides.

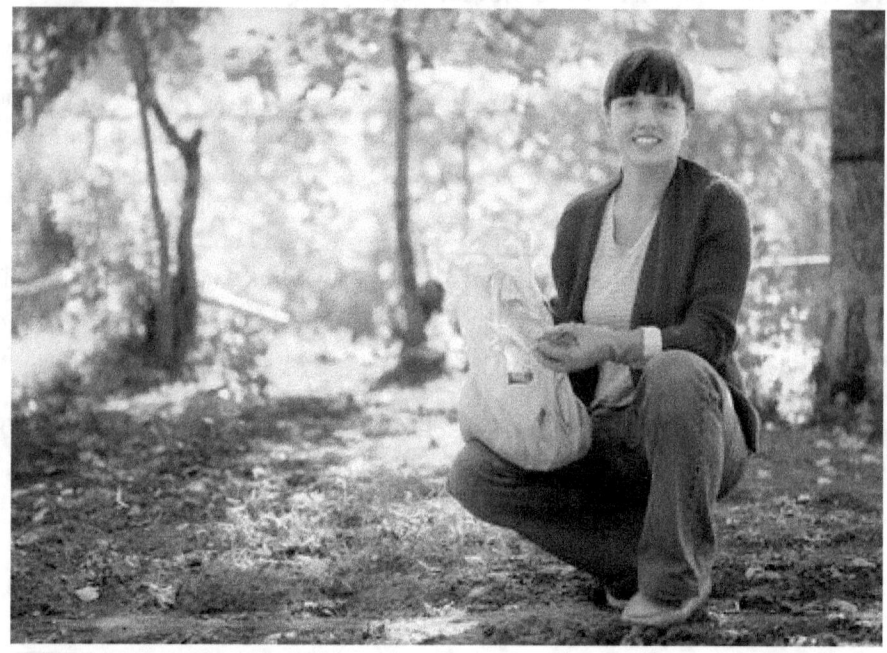

Use natural fertilizers as far as possible, while growing organic foods

No use of artificial food coloring added to the final product.

No use of chemical preservatives in the final product. Did you know that in the 21st century, the high sodium intake of children can be blamed on food firms? In 2004, research was done on how much of this food was taken between home and school. The answer was a whopping USD350 million! You can imagine how much it is today with more and more sodium-based junk foods coming into the market.

Is it surprising that so many children are suffering from obesity? The chemical preservatives, high sodium, food coloring and other products to make these food items last longer and look more attractive, are important factors, bent on ruining the health of your kids.

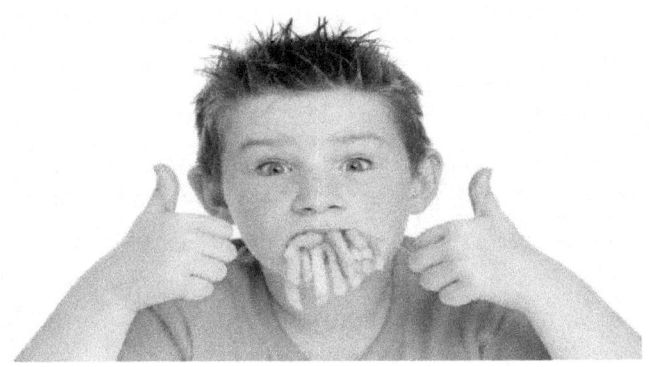

The only artificial preservatives, which should be allowed in organic food are sodium nitrates and nitrites, which are approved for use in curing bacon and ham.

It has been found out that many countries use artificial growth promoters in the rearing of animals. These include harmful hormones. Organic food, especially meat reared for eating, definitely does not include growth promoters, but those animals are fed on natural food items.

I went visiting some relatives living in a desert area and was astonished at the delicious flavor of the meat cooked and fed to us. A little bit of judicial inquiry told me that it was not the spices which made that meat so tasty, but the food on which the animal was fed. The land was arid. These animals could only eat herbs growing in that desert land, and drink the water available in waterholes.

This totally pesticide free diet flavored the meat in such a manner, that every bit of it was exported abroad, especially to the Middle East. The locals got to eat it on very special and festive occasions. And it was a gourmet treat.

Now that was hundred percent totally organic meat. Our ancestors ate it, millenniums ago. They did not eat food contaminated with chemicals, artificial preservatives and growth promoters.

Organic meat should also be raised without the animals being fed antibiotics. Drugs should never be used as growth enhancers or prophylactics.

Do you know that the major contributing factor for mad cow disease, which caused their brains to deteriorate, and the complete failure of the nervous system was based on feeding cows *animal protein*? You did not know that, did you?

This is the best kept secret, your farmers and your government and the press has hidden from you.

According to the Wikipedia, Indian cow breeds were resistant to this disease. What people do not know is that in the Indian subcontinent, Indian cows are definitely *not fed meat*. They are fed hay, grain, and greens. There is no question of feeding a farm bred animal chopped meat, because apart from it being considered anathema and sacrilege, no farmer would ever think of such a silly thing to do in order to supposedly improve the quality of meat and its quantity.

So organic meat means making sure that the meat you eat has not – in its own turn – been fed on meat. Farm Animals are basically vegetarian. Changing their diet patterns and habits is going to destroy them.

Take this as an example and moral story for human beings too. We are naturally herbivores and have learned to be carnivores. But when we start being omnivores, we may find that having a detrimental effect on the general state of our health.

Organic food also means that the food you eat is not genetically modified.

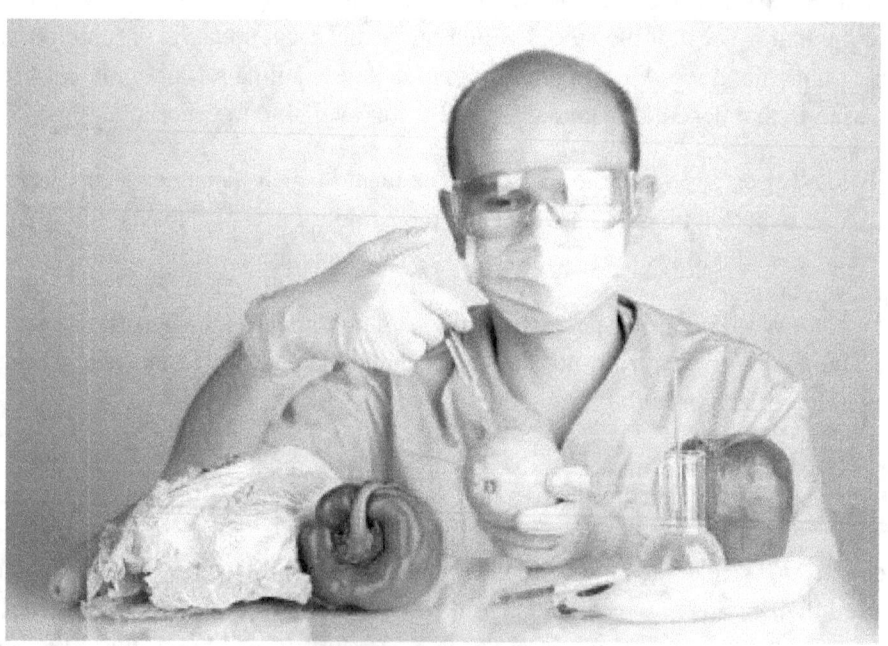

Believe it or not, scientists are still experimenting with growth enhancers, not bothering much about the longer-term harmful effects, they are going to have on the general health of the consumers. And the governments of many countries are not taking steps in preventing or stopping such experimentations.

Pesticides in Food

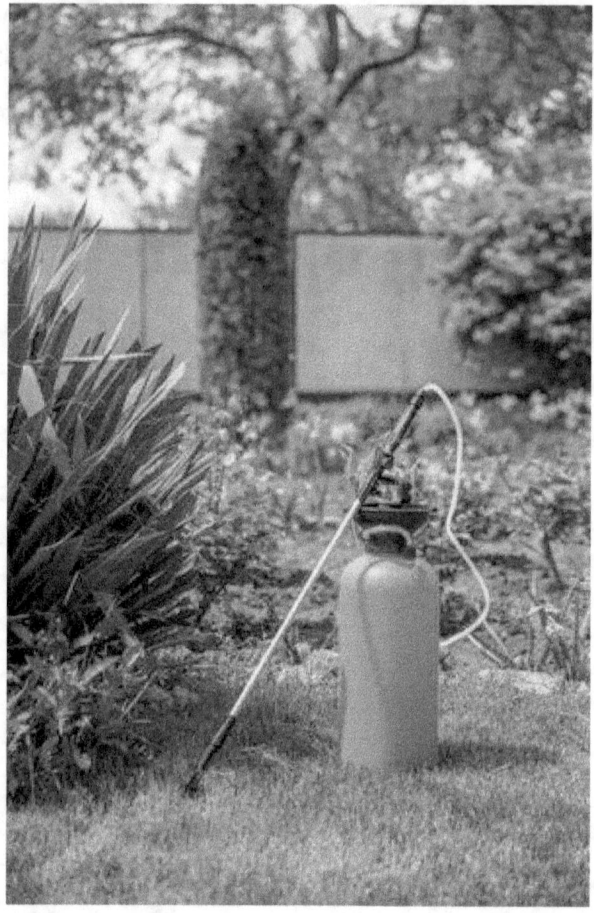

These pesticides not only pollute and contaminate your garden, but they are also a potential health hazard.

Did you know that 27% of all the foods which you consume consist of pesticides in some form or the other? It is a well-documented fact that 33 – 43% of the fruit and vegetables you eat have been contaminated with pesticides.

Even 11% of branded baby foods, which you should have believed to be safe, have residues of pesticide in them.

The cocktail of these pesticide residues accumulating in a baby through the foods he eats is naturally going to have a future long-term bad effect on his health.

On the other hand, organically grown foods are not subjected to DDT, antibiotics, genetic engineering and other potentially harmful chemicals and practices.

Animal manure is actually in use in both organic and conventional farming. High organic standards specify scientific composting procedures, in modern day organic farms. But in many parts of the world, where traditional organic food growing methods are still being used in order to produce food, the old methods of composting are still being used and the product utilized as an excellent natural fertilizer for the soil.

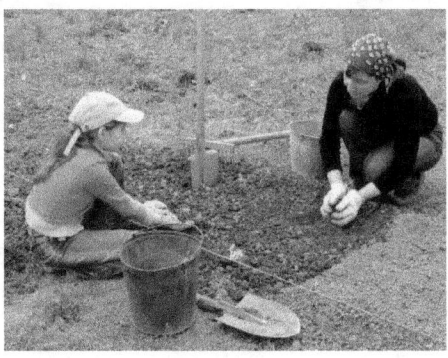

Organic compost, added to the soil before sowing is going to give you a healthy, natural product yield.

Organic Junk Foods...

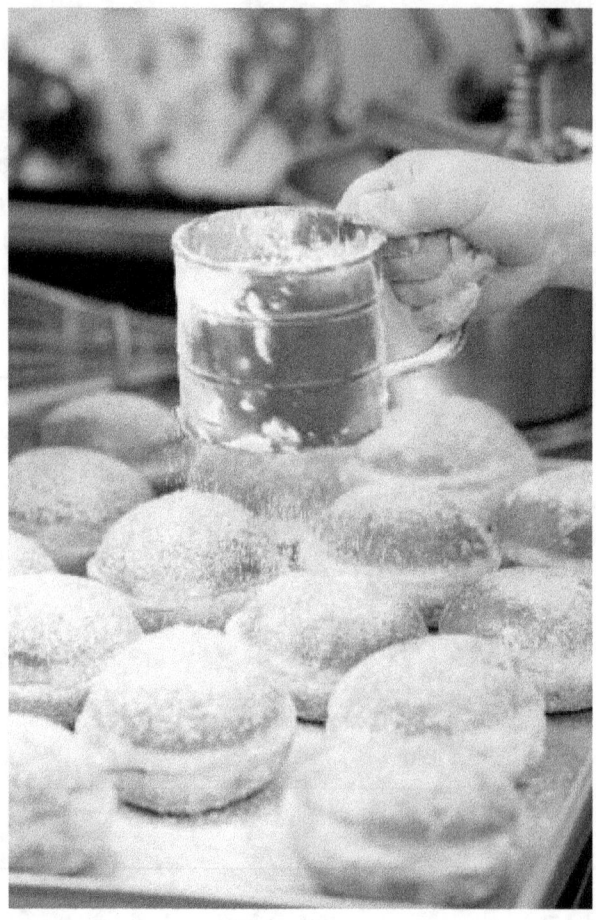

These doughnuts may be organic, but do you think they are healthy? Is not the powdered sugar being sifted over them, a bit too much?

Now that the word has gone forth, that eat organic is going to be the norm of the day, is it a wonder that many brand names have jumped on the word "Organic"as a magical advertising keyword, just like "Natural. "

That is why you have organic doughnuts and organic foodstuffs made up of organic sugar, and organic white flour. Now, are they healthy? I do not think so. Sugar in itself is not healthy, be it organic or nonorganic. White flour is refined flour, and refined flour, even if it is organic is not nutritional nor is it healthy.

So here you are, your child is eating organic junk food.

Packaged foods provide a large and high profit margin and that is why manufacturers, jumping on this organic bandwagon have begun to use this word indiscriminately in order to entice parents into buying their products. This is misleading the consumer of a high order.

The advertising style is so attractive and seductive, that you assuage your conscience, when you are buying organic sweets and organic doughnuts, because you have persuaded yourself that they are healthy items. You know that they are not healthy because of their sweet content. So why are you ruining your health and your childrens' healths with food items sold to you by unscrupulous marketeers?

This is when you are going to read the label. Just looking at the word organic on the label and putting it right in your shopping basket is definitely not a sensible idea. Just because the word is written there, along with Natural, it does not mean that it is going to be healthy.

There are many brands of supposedly organic cereals, which have plenty of sugar and salt added to them.

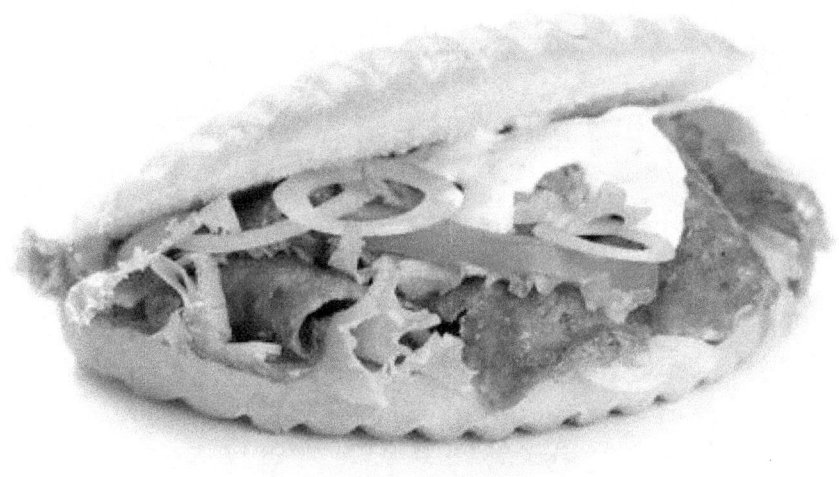

This does not need to be made up of fried items. Use fresh vegetables and broiled or grilled bacon, in between whole-wheat bread.

Look for brands which are additive free and low on the sodium and sugar content. Some really good frozen convenience food companies like Whole Earth Foods – can give you a wide range of organic additive free healthy foods. This is a British company and is slowly and steadily making its name and reputation of healthy organic packed, canned, and bottled organic foods.

http://wholeearthfoods.com/

Taste and Nutritional Benefits

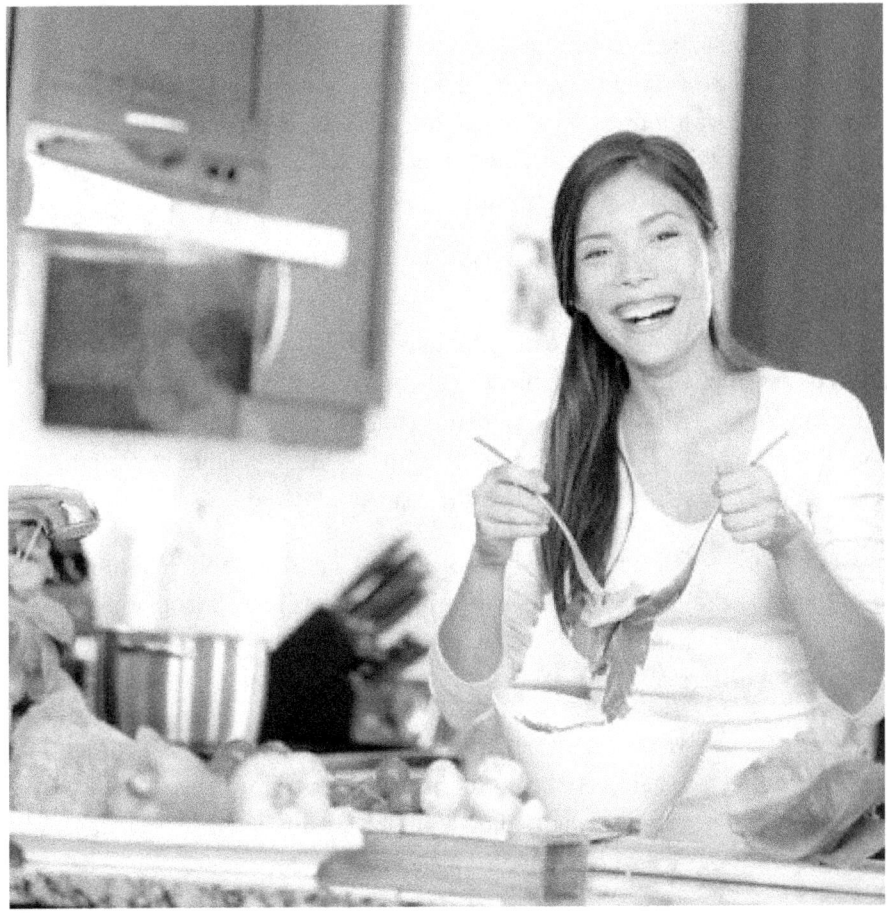

She appreciates good healthy food.

I fondly remember my American cousin coming home, to our native heath, and demanding lots and lots of fresh farm grown vegetables for breakfast, lunch and dinner. She found the meals delicious and wondered why those lettuces in the produce section of her supermarket did not quite taste the same?

When I, [Bender of joys that I am,] took her around the farm and showed her the stinking cow dung heap, which was used to fertilize the soil, she gave me a "why the @#$%^ did you need to disillusion me, could not you have left well alone?" look.

And I felt that she was going to deck me a juicy one when I burbled, "that is the stuff which makes the food so tasty."

Many people are squeamish about the fact that the natural manure which is used to fertilize the land is stinking animal manure and rotting compost. But, that is the traditional farming procedure, which has been used in many parts of the world for centuries. Natural Pesticides include neem oil , bougainvillea leaves, cayenne pepper, etc. mixed with water.

The yield produces delicious natural, non-toxic, healthy vegetables which have not been subjected to the toxins of the 21st century. But then anybody – like my cousin – who has been used to eating foods which have been genetically modified, or which have been subject to chemicals, pesticides and other nonorganic and potentially lethal foodstuffs may not understand that these items are used for the protection of the plant. And the produce's natural taste and its innate health content are sacrificed on the road side.

Many newspapers have articles, which broadcast a belief that organic foods taste better. In a way they are right, because your taste buds have got so attuned to eating genetically enhanced foods that any sort of natural produce foodstuff is going to taste different.

They have a lower water content and that is why they are going to hold the shape better, when they are being cooked. So this is the reason why, you "feel"that they taste better, especially when other vegetables, which have not been grown organically turn mushy with the addition of a little water.

Organic chickens are definitely going to taste better, because they are eating nutritional and natural stuffs. Their living conditions are also marginally better, because there are out in the farm, foraging for animal protein for themselves. All this exercise also means that the meat is less fatty, stronger tasting, and not so stringy.

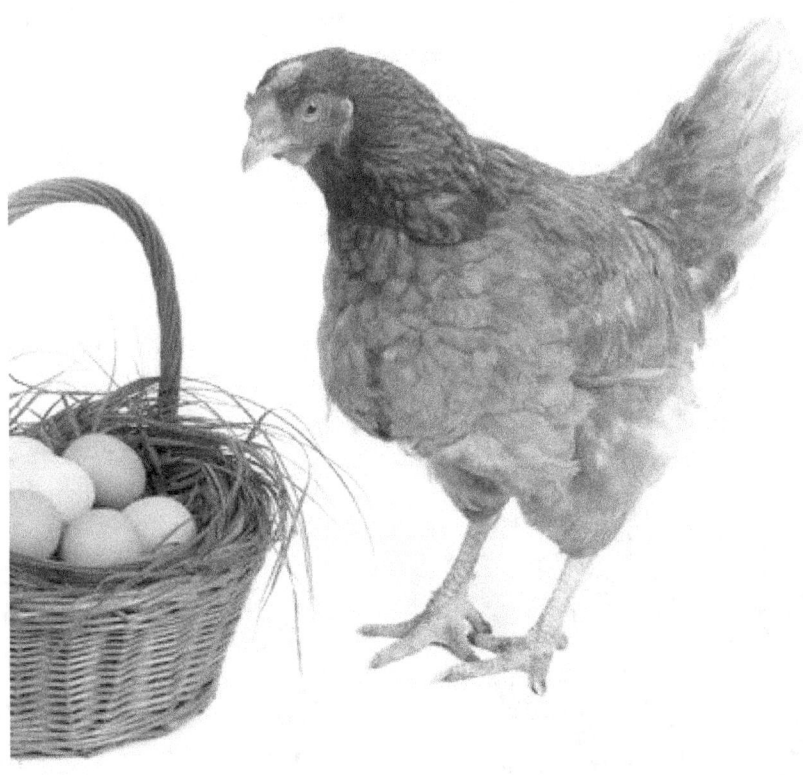

I still remember my father raising chickens for the table, when we were kids. Every morning, they were given full permission to go out in the garden and forage for themselves. Along with that, they used to get a food supplement of powdered wheat bran husk, dried fishmeal/offal, broken corn seeds, and groundnut oil cakes from which the oil had been extracted.

I remember seeing him mix these together in a bowl, every afternoon, and the birds making a beeline for him, especially when they knew that they were going to have fishmeal. I also remember one particular bird –Kook– who just could not resist picking the best pieces of dried fish in the bowl, even while he was mixing and her beak met with the back of his hand the number of times on different occasions. So we children were asked to pick her up, to her great indignation.

Believe it or not, hens can make their displeasure felt by using very bad language, but then when Kook saw that the others did not approach the bowl while he was mixing, and she was the first one placed in front of the bowl after the mixing procedure was done, she began to be very pleased with the proceedings and watched his activities with a very bright eye, clucking softly to herself.

After all, this fresh meal was being mixed for her to taste first, before other birds could eat. So they are definitely not bird – wits. This was also when we began to learn about bird psychology, at a tender age!

The eggs produced from these birds which were white Leghorns were almost as delicious as those produced by native breeds. And the meat was flavorsome, strong tasting, and amazingly tender and juicy. This was due to the fishmeal and the organic food protein scrounged during the daily free ranging in the garden.

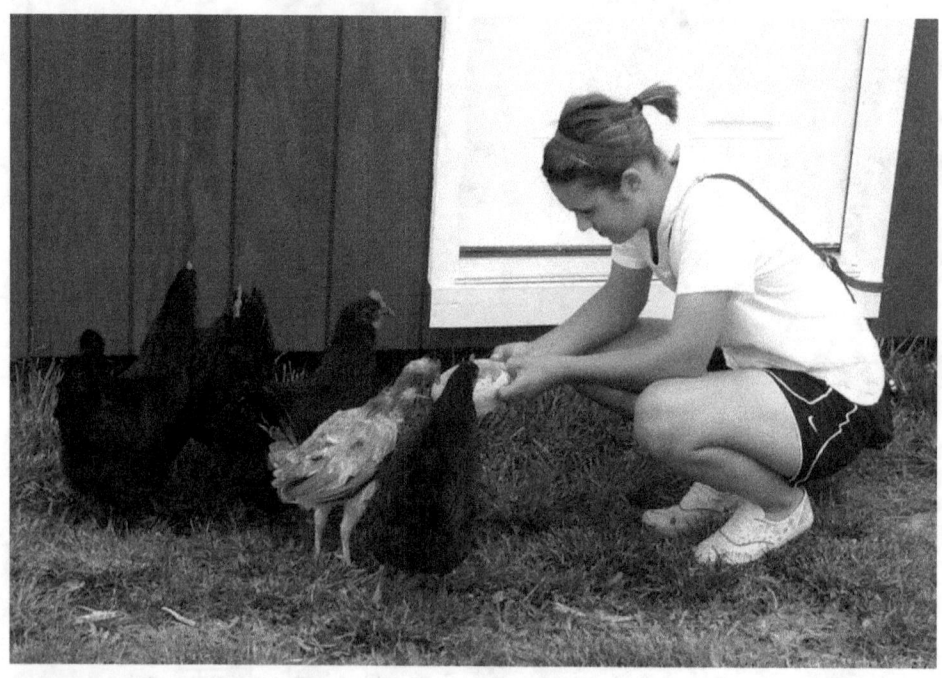

Cost Factor

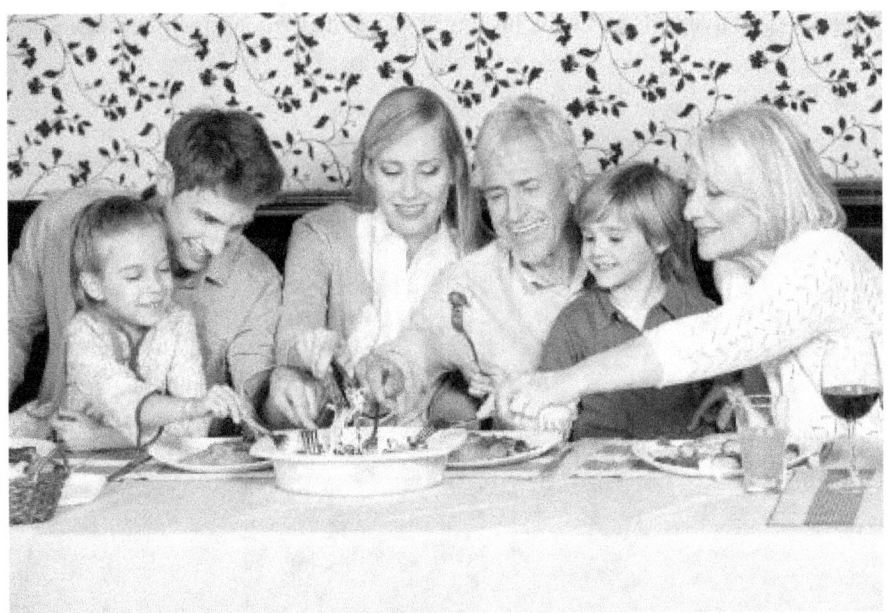

Good healthy food does not need to be expensive and exotic

I was surprised to see that the cost factor for organic food abroad is considerably higher than nonorganic food. The explanation given is that the yield in an organic farm is lesser than on a nonorganic farm. I do not consider that to be a logical explanation, especially when the farming technologies in the West are more sophisticated and much more advanced than those being followed in the East.

Organic farming, the traditional way is definitely the way in which fruit and vegetables and meat is being raised in many parts of the world, especially in Asia, the Middle East, and all these products are being exported to the West. So what I think is that people are being made to believe that organic produce is something exotic, and special. That is why they have to pay a higher price in order to buy anything organic.

This is a marketing strategy being used by supermarkets, who sell these produce at higher rates. So I would suggest going to local farms, where they are producing organic foodstuffs. Get your fresh produce from their farm directly.

This means that you will need to cook from scratch. This also means that you are going to be cutting down conventional fast foods and ready to cook foods. Try buying inexpensive pulses, beans, grains and greens, fruit and vegetables.

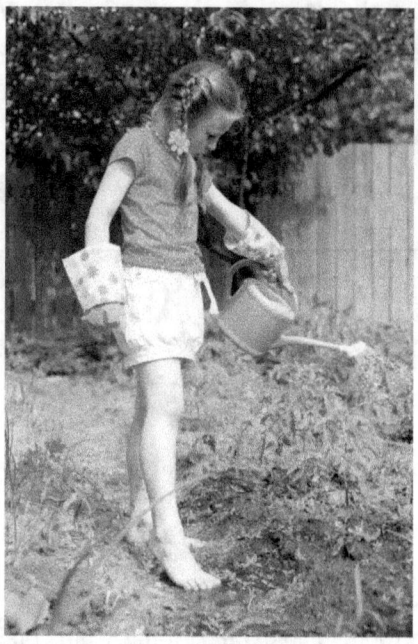

Children learning to garden at a young age are going to appreciate eating the food that they have grown themselves.

No Chemicals

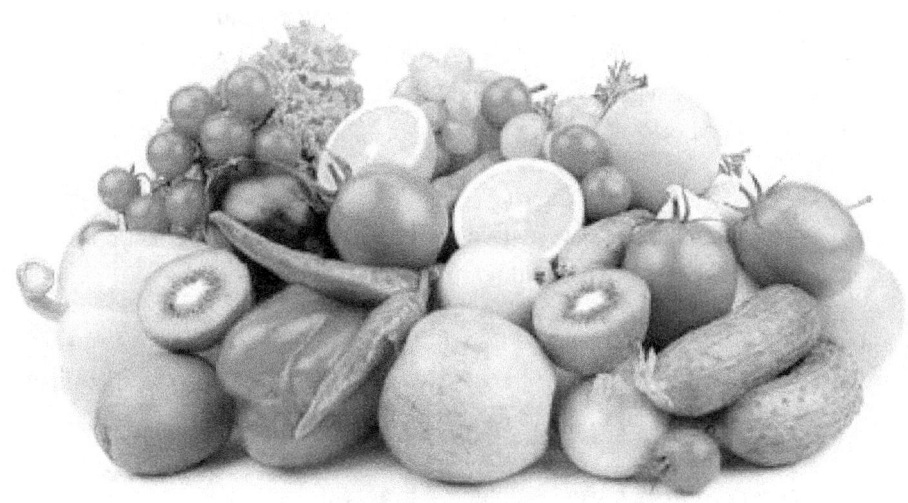

I speak now of a relative whose farm is still being worked on traditional methods. Even in this day and age of pesticides and chemical products, she still advocates the use of old time natural fertilizers and natural pesticides. [That was the farm which was inspected by my over – sophisticated and used – to – modern – farming methods – and – technology cousin, to her great dismay.]

Her harvest goes straight in the local market. Every Tuesday, local buyers make a beeline for her stall. And when other farmers found out that her produce was still being grown organically, and asked to taste her produce, many of them gave up chemical pesticides and chemical fertilizers. So you can consider this to be a local unspoken revolution, of eat organic, protect your health, save the soil campaign.

She is now in her 60s. Her father is in his 90s. The food the family eats is supplied directly from the farm to her kitchen. The whole family is considered to be the healthiest in the neighborhood. QED.

She is teaching the people of our area, most of them with an agricultural and farming background, how to say no, to chemicals. You as a consumer can get chemicals out of the lives of your children by buying organic food whenever possible. Organic milk, vegetables, fruit and meat is particularly important in the initial stages of a child's growth.

When we were young, somebody asked my father why we children were just given chicken and red meat in small quantities to eat up to the age of six and seven, and it was only when we were eight or so, that we were allowed to eat red meat in the form of pork sausages, bacon, ham, salami and mutton in normal helpings.

As babies and youngsters, we were given only one small piece of bacon for breakfast with eggs so that we could learn how to digest it.

His answer was that from babyhood to childhood, a child needs proper nutrition in order to grow healthy. His digestive system needs to learn how to adapt itself to easily digestible food and then to food which is a little hard to digest. By the time we were eight or so, we could have hard to digest red meat in larger quantities, because now we were reaching our growth spurt stage, when we needed plenty of protein-based food.

And both of us kids hit around 6 Feet, as adults, in happy, healthy bodies, because of this good eating habit. [You could say genes also had something to do with this particular growth spurt, but a diet all through the first 14 years of our lives totally based on garden produce, and organic food can be considered to be responsible for our healthy digestive systems, very strong immunity system and lots of strength and energy.]

Healthy Bodies and Healthy Minds

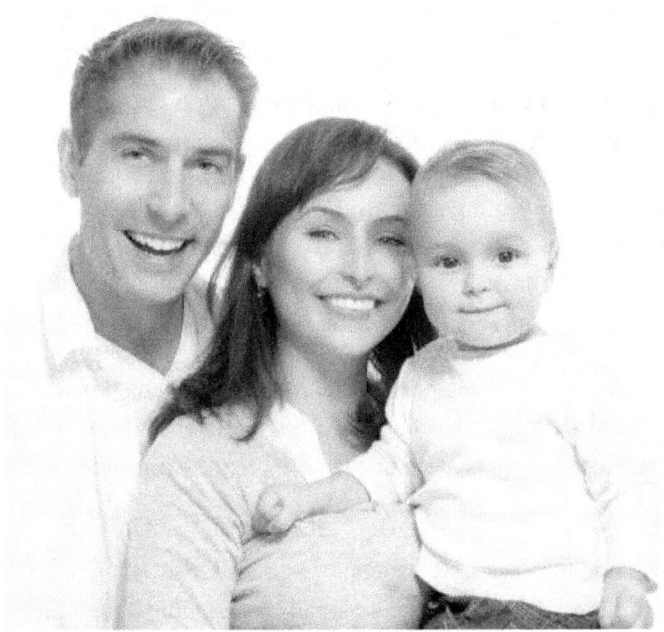

Besides, good nutritious food, we were not allowed to sit idle throughout the day. Apart from the exercise, we had at school, playing games, we had more than 3 to 4 hours of muscle building activities promoting tissue growth. This included walking, running, jumping, and generally making lots of noises as supposedly adventurous explorers in our garden or in the jungles surrounding Our Base.

This energetic frame of mind, especially a happy child shows that he is getting a good, healthy nutritious diet, and in large quantities. The end result was, we came home hungry as little wolves, finished everything on our plates and got our regular 10 – 11 hours sleep – like – a – baby rest from 9 to 7.

The result was that the only time we went to doctors was to get ourselves bandaged because we had fallen down and hurt ourselves. We never were given drugs. In fact, the only medicine in our house was the headache remedy Crocin, and that was for dad, – because he was a grown-up and he had headaches – and not for us!

The only time we fell ill was when we came to the cities during our holidays. That is when we caught measles and mumps and chickenpox! And our grandfather advocated that we be fed fresh chicken soup, instead of being given antibiotics, which would harm our natural resistance power to fight off diseases.

This outdoor activity gave us plenty of scope to continue the same adventures and exercises as we grew, because we were used to them as children. How many children today are encouraged to go outside and just play? They would rather sit inside a stuffy room and watch TV or play video games.

So remember, if you are giving your children, drugs and medicines indiscriminately, because the doctor says so, stop that immediately. You are ruining his natural immunity system. But you say, my child needs this medicine, because he is subject to infections, and flu and fever and allergies.

Stop and think. Your child was born basically healthy. His health began to deteriorate, as he got exposed to chemical treatments around the garden and the house, flea treatments for pets, contaminated water and air, wood treatments, and garden pesticides.

Childrens parks and playing fields are sprayed regularly with pesticides. If this is being followed in your town, go to your local counsel and check their spraying schedule. Do not allow your child to go in that park for the next four days, after a schedule has been implemented.

Instead, take him to another park, where he can breathe fresh chemical free air.

Remember not to wrap any fatty foods such as cheese, or bacon in plastic wrapping. Plastic wrapping leaches phenolic compounds. Instead, ask your butcher to wrap up the meat in waxed paper.

Healthy Eating Outdoors

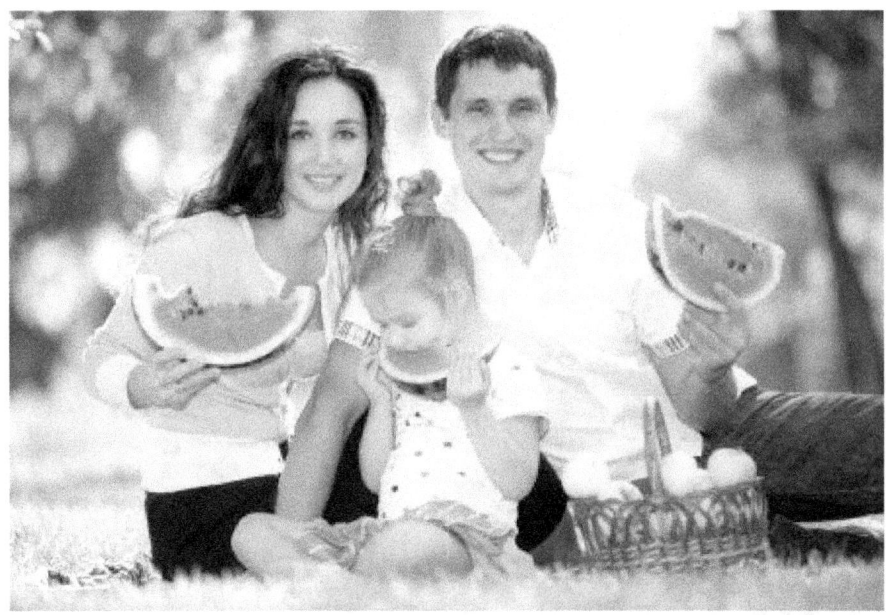

Children love eating outdoors, especially in picnics, and barbecues. That can give you a good opportunity to use plenty of herbs, whole wheat bread, organic meat, sausages and bagels, tortilla wraps, and other different types of breads.

You can use up a large number of leftovers such as roasted vegetables, by combining them with rice and tossed with a vinaigrette. Or you can mix chopped cucumber, spring onions, a clove of garlic tomato, fresh mint and cheese with boiled porridge or couscous and add your preferred herbs and spices along with some dressing.

Use yogurt dips in which you have added cayenne, pepper, salt and a choice of your own favorite herbs, including mint and parsley.

Finger food in outdoor eating means chance of cheese, and right tomatoes with French bread, small baked quiches, sliced vegetables, bunches of fruit like grapes chopped up and mixed with other fruits in a fruit salad, and a teaspoonful of lemon juice, and boiled chicken. Just pull off pieces of boiled chicken from the main chicken frame and eat with tomatoes, radishes, or with a little bit of salt sprinkled on it.

Do not deprive your child of sweets, by saying that it is not organic eating and too many sweets is not healthy. Try raisins, berries, watermelons, citrus fruits, banana bread, banana chips, muffins are all tasty, especially when they are eaten outdoors.

Different Food Textures

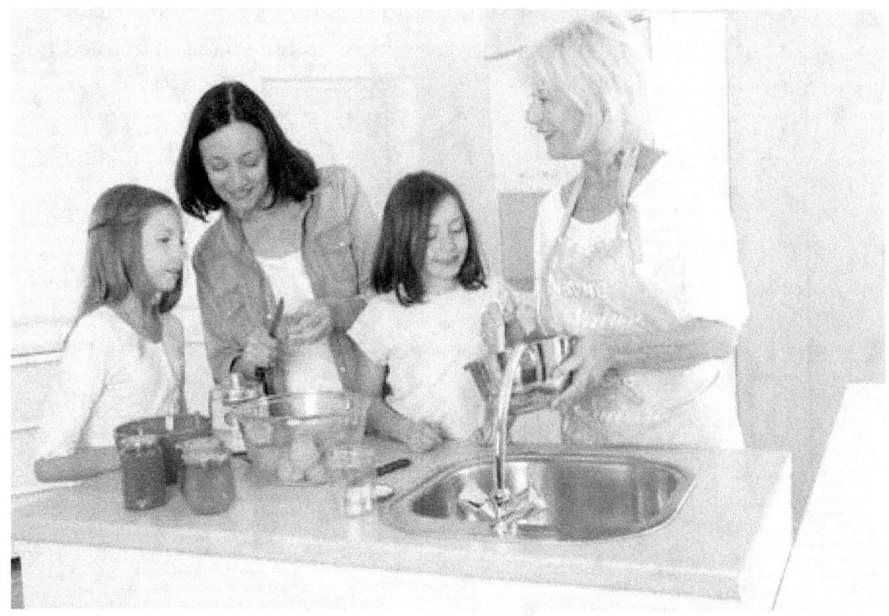

Start your children young in the appreciation of good food.

One of my friends enjoyed eating pineapple chunks with pieces of sardine. When children experiment with different foodstuffs and textures at a very young age, they are developing their own taste buds. I do not mind eating crisply fried spicy ladies finger, with plenty of chilies and chopped onions, put in a bowlful of yogurt. I do not allow the yogurt or the ladies' finger to get soggy. And this combination tastes really delicious with crisply Wok fried rice with vegetables and pieces of meat.

You can make meat kebabs for barbecuing outdoors, by interspersing chunks of lamb and chicken, with fruit chunks of pineapple, apple, and even pears. You can also use onions, yellow peppers, baby sweet corn, mushrooms and marinated tofu.

Here are some different marinade combinations for your barbecue.

Mustard, honey and olive oil, which is excellent for lamb chops and sausages.

Onion, tomato, red pepper, garlic, olive oil and paprika mixture for meat.

Yogurt, garlic, lemon, olive oil, and mint – our traditional family marinade recipe, with lots of cayenne pepper and salt added, and the meat marinated for 24 hours to tenderize it in the yogurt.

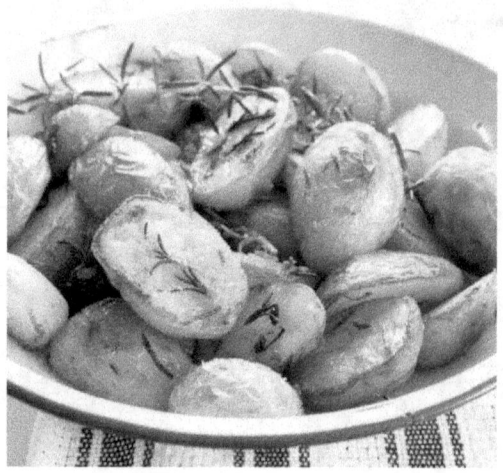

Olive oil with herbs added to it, like sage, rosemary and garlic.

Safety Tips While Eating Outdoors

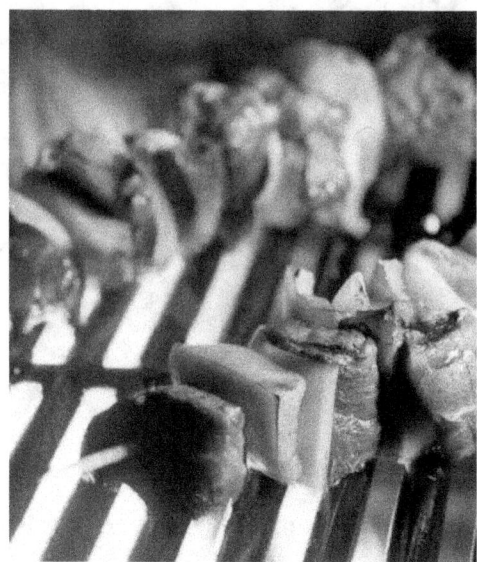

You may want to look at these safety tips, especially when you are eating outdoors in the summer. Summer is the time when temperatures rise. This also means bacterial growth is going to be more prolific than normal. So if you are putting meat stuff in your car, in an area which gets heated, make sure that you cook the meat at the picnic spot for a long while, and at a high temperature. This is going to prevent food poisoning.

Better still, I would suggest placing milk, fish, meat, fresh dips, sauces and cheese, which you are taking along with you in an outdoor barbecue or picnic in a cool box with ice packs. You may want to cook any dishes which you are packing for your picnic, thoroughly beforehand.

Shellfish, cheeses, and mayonnaise are particularly vulnerable to high temperature so it may be best to avoid taking them for picnics, unless of course you are sure you are keeping them cool.

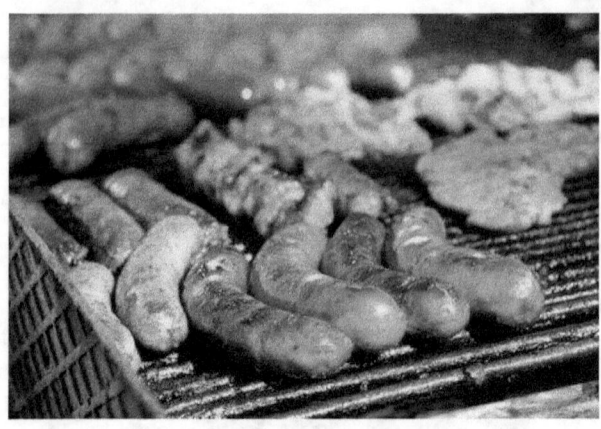

Make sure the meat is cooked properly and at a high temperature, before eating it.

Make sure that any barbecued meat is cooked properly. Food that is burnt outside, and raw inside is not only unhealthy to eat, but it also is an aesthetically not so pleasing sight. To make sure that this does not happen, check that your barbecue is at the right temperature for cooking. The flames should have died down. The coals should be glowing, and the tray should not be very close or too far away from the coals.

Cut the meat up into small enough pieces to ensure that the center is cooked sufficiently and keep turning the pieces so that all the sides are cooked properly. Make sure that you test the meat after it has been done by cutting into its center before serving.

Children outdoors, especially in the summer need plenty of juices in order to keep them properly dehydrated, especially when they are going to be running about in the sun.

Never give an overheated child an icy cold drink. I remember as a child, running to the fridge, drenched with sweat, and being stopped by my grandmother. She would tell me to sit down, and a drink would be given to me only when my grandmother had inspected me properly and declared "the sweat has dried now. You can now have cold water to drink."

Remember that your own thirst gauge is no measure about how thirsty a child is going to feel, and when, and how often, because you are an adult and he is a child, much smaller in body size. So have an individual bottle of water for each child, and they can swig a couple of mouthfuls whenever they feel thirsty.

In the same manner we were not allowed to shower when we came indoors, overheated and all sweaty and grimy. We were made to sit down, relax for about 10 minutes, in a cool temperature under the fan and then allowed to go have a shower.

Conclusion

This book introduces the concept of healthy eating for children along with organic food. A little bit of sensible education about food, and encouraging your children to eat nutritious food is going to make your children healthy and happy.

Good eating habits, along with common sense tips can make food fun instead of it being just some boring, bland stuff which you need to eat. A change in lifestyle, which incorporates the new family culture of enjoying food together is going to make for a memorable and healthy childhood. Food is interesting, food is delicious food is also fun. As long as you are eating it with convivial company which means friends, and family members. Also discovering new cuisines is an adventure, if you have not tried it out before.

So for people who think shopping for food is a bore, food preparation is a boring chore, eating is something which needs to be gotten out of the way as quickly as possible, avoiding ingredients in recipes which you do not know how to cook as they might mess up the dish, and other such trivial excuses, is not it time that you began to think about the effect this lack of proper nutrition is having on your child?

Do you know that the attitude of parents towards food is going to affect their children's view of eating and health? Many parents in the USA or in the UK have their own ideas of what foods are healthy, and which are not, as a result of their own particular attitudes towards dieting. So if they do not eat it, their children will not get an opportunity to eat it.

On the other hand, moms in Italy and Spain are more interested in feeding their children, and feeding them well. When they convey their own pleasure in cooking, they are instilling a positive attitude in their children towards eating and thus providing a direct link to good health.

So encourage the appreciation of good food by involving your children in discovering new foods, and taking an interest in how new dishes are made.

Good and healthy eating is your child's birthright. So teach them to appreciate this pleasurable activity.

Live long and prosper!

Author Bio

Dueep Jyot Singh is a Management and IT Professional who managed to gather Postgraduate qualifications in Management and English and Degrees in Science, French and Education while pursuing different enjoyable career options like being an hospital administrator, IT,SEO and HRD Database Manager/ trainer, movie , radio and TV scriptwriter, theatre artiste and public speaker, lecturer in French, Marketing and Advertising, ex-Editor of Hearts On Fire (now known as Solstice) Books Missouri USA, advice columnist and cartoonist, publisher and Aviation School trainer, ex- moderator on Medico.in, banker, student councilor ,travelogue writer … among other things!

One fine morning, she decided that she had enough of killing herself by Degrees and went back to her first love -- writing. It's more enjoyable! She already has 48 published academic and 14 fiction- in- different- genre books under her belt.

When she is not designing websites or making Graphic design illustrations for clients , she is browsing through old bookshops hunting for treasures, of which she has an enviable collection – including R.L. Stevenson, O.Henry, Dornford Yates, Maurice Walsh, De Maupassant, Victor Hugo, Sapper, C.N. Williamson, "Bartimeus" and the crown of her collection- Dickens "The Old Curiosity Shop," and so on… Just call her "Renaissance Woman") - collecting herbal remedies, acting like Universal Helping Hand/Agony Aunt, or escaping to her dear mountains for a bit of exploring, collecting herbs and plants and trekking.

1. Amazon.com
2. Barnes and Noble
3. Itunes
4. Kobo
5. Smashwords
6. Google Play Books

Check out some of the other JD-Biz Publishing books

Gardening Series on Amazon

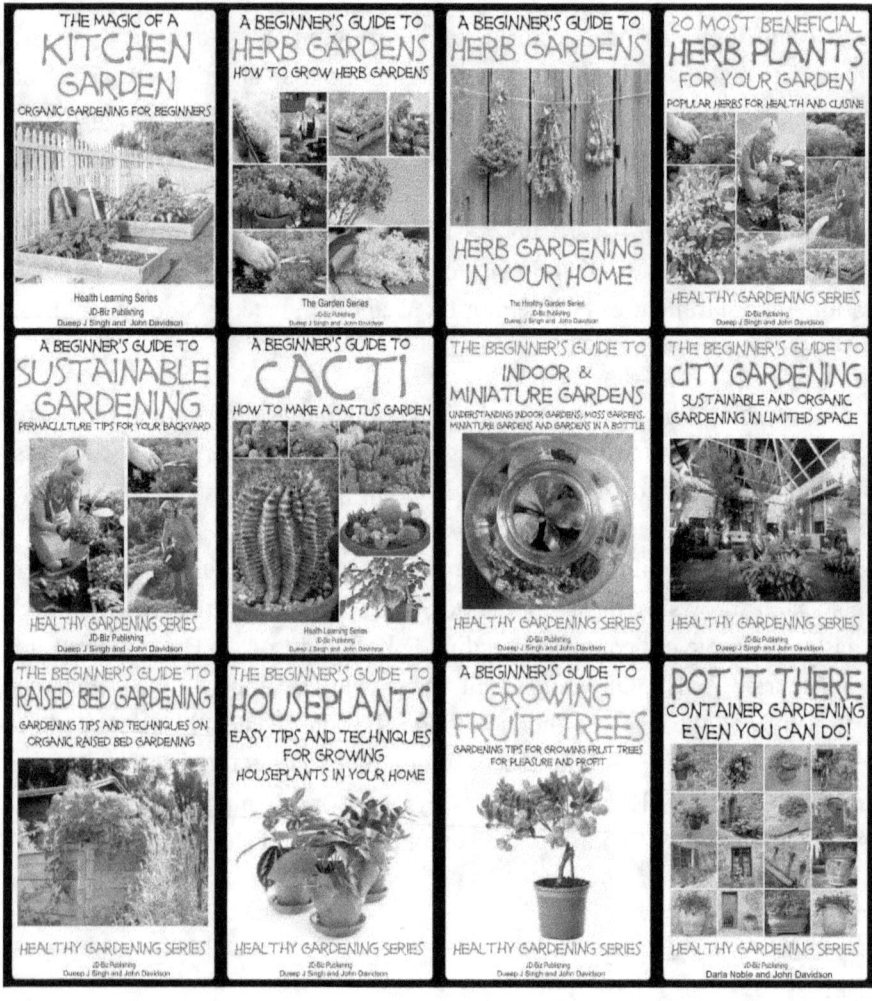

Health Learning Series

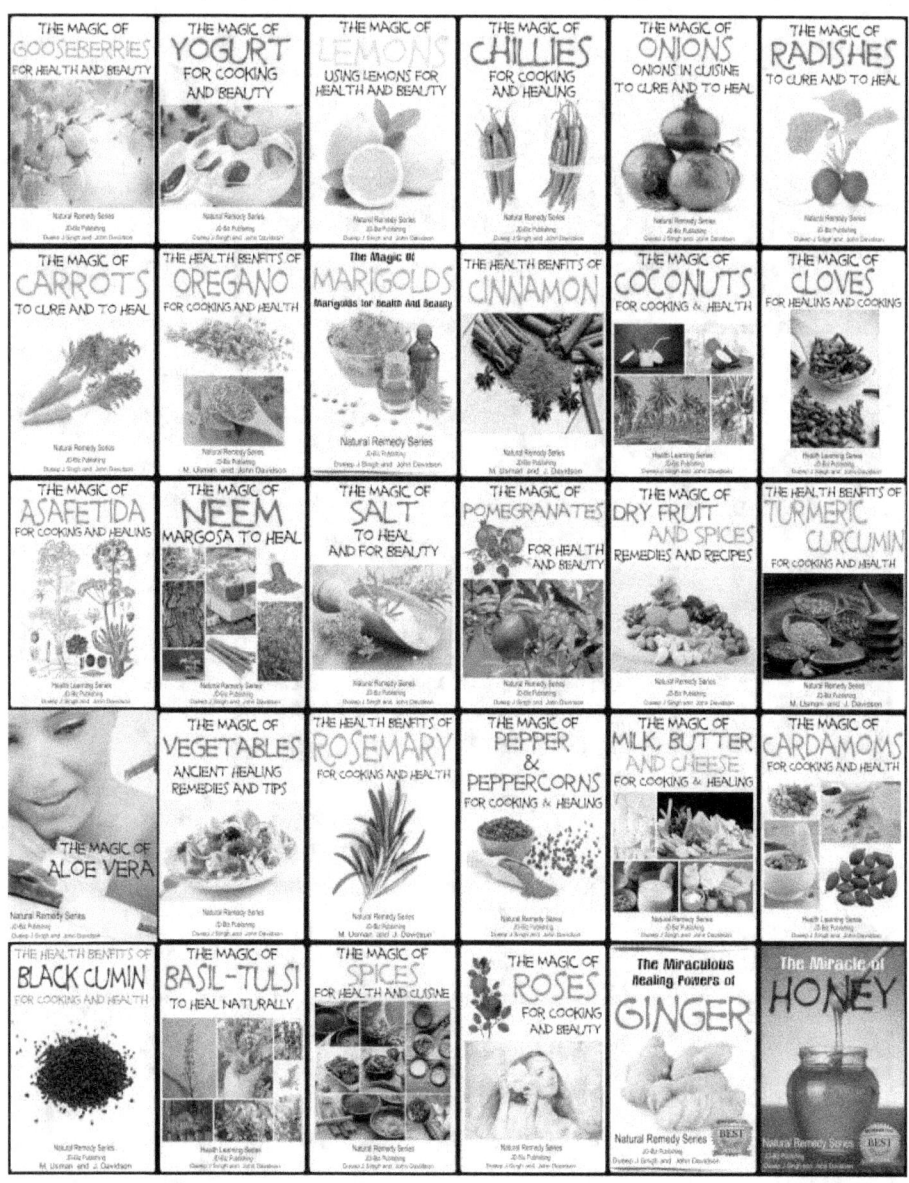

Country Life Books

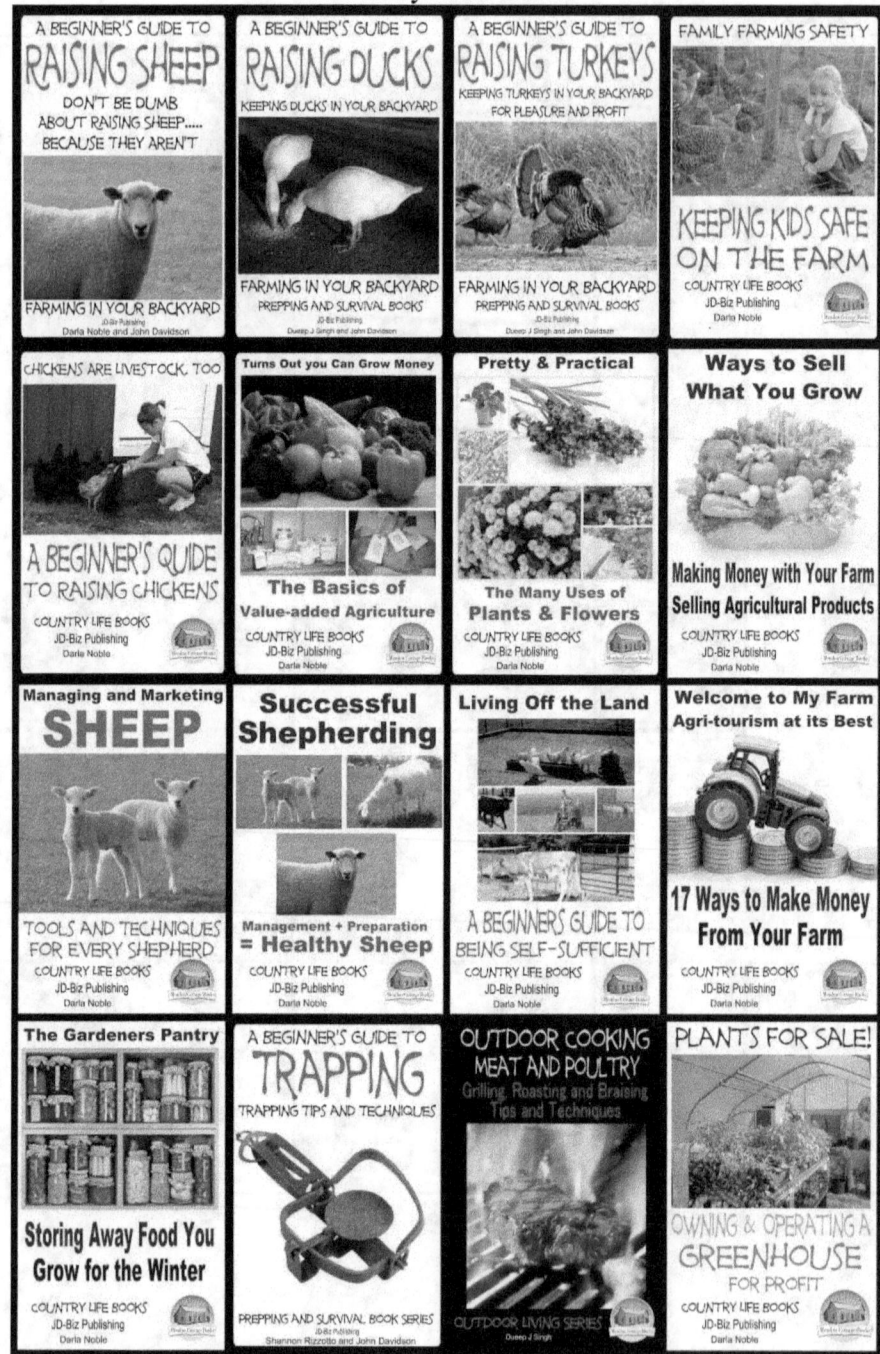

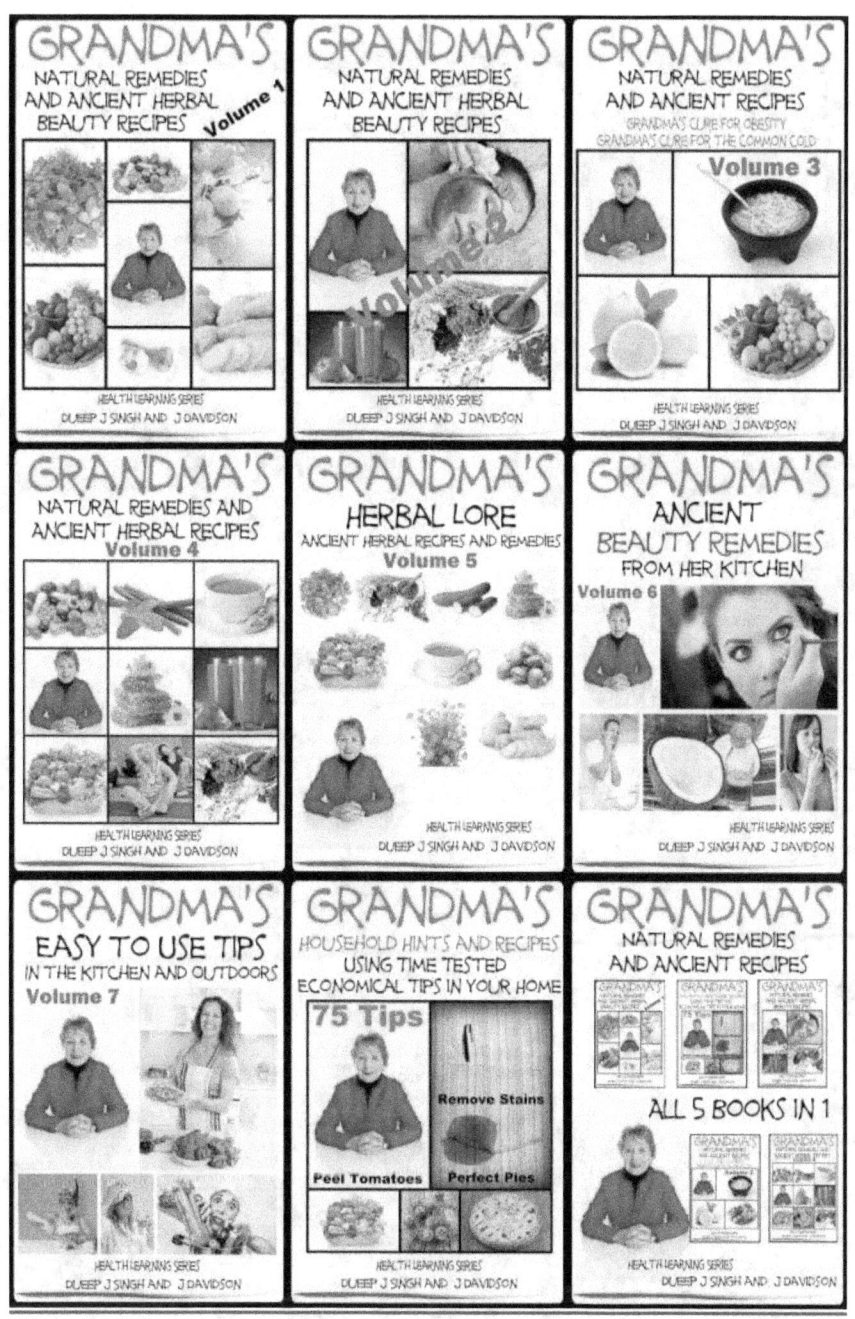

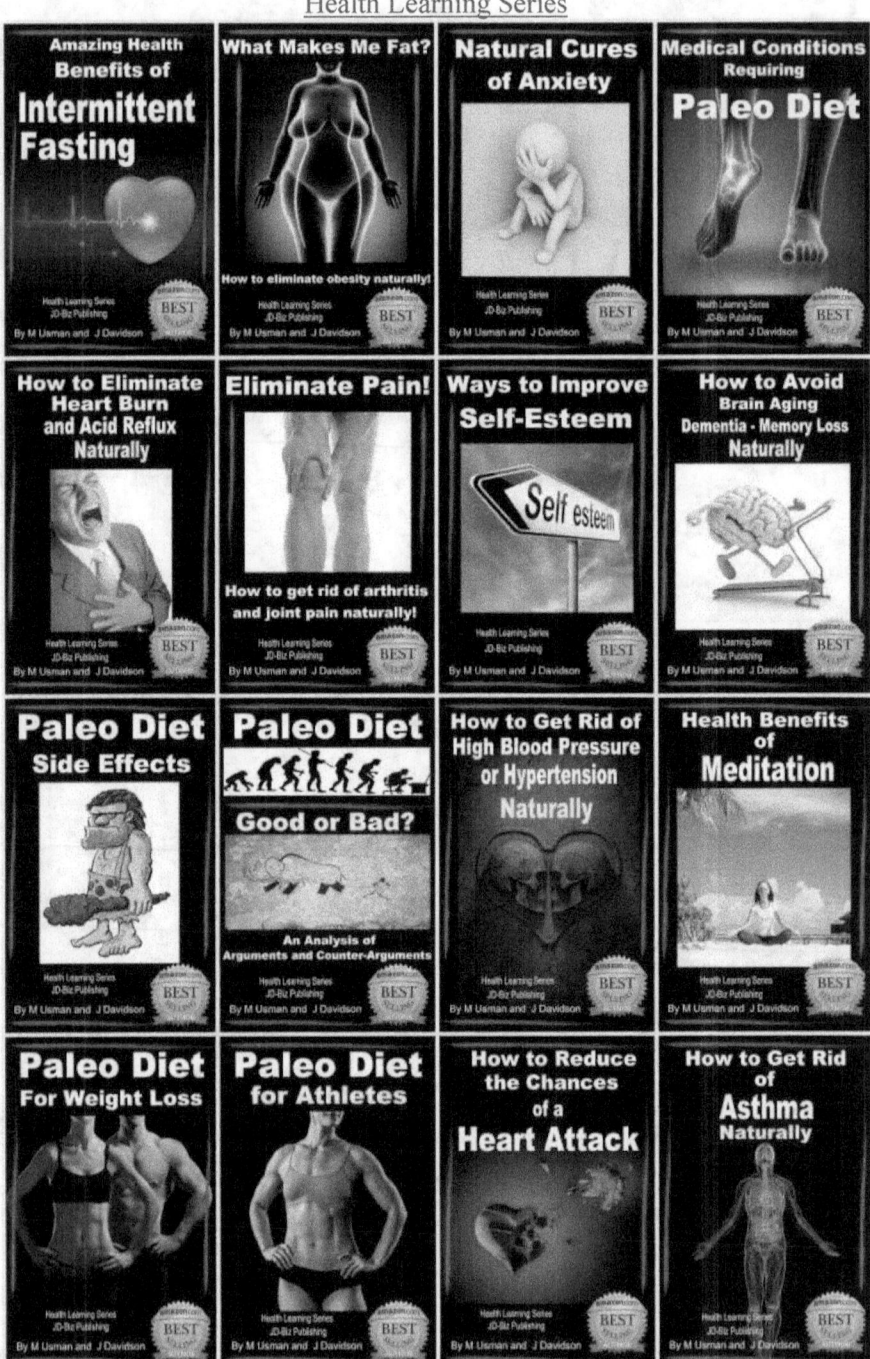

Amazing Animal Book Series

Learn To Draw Series

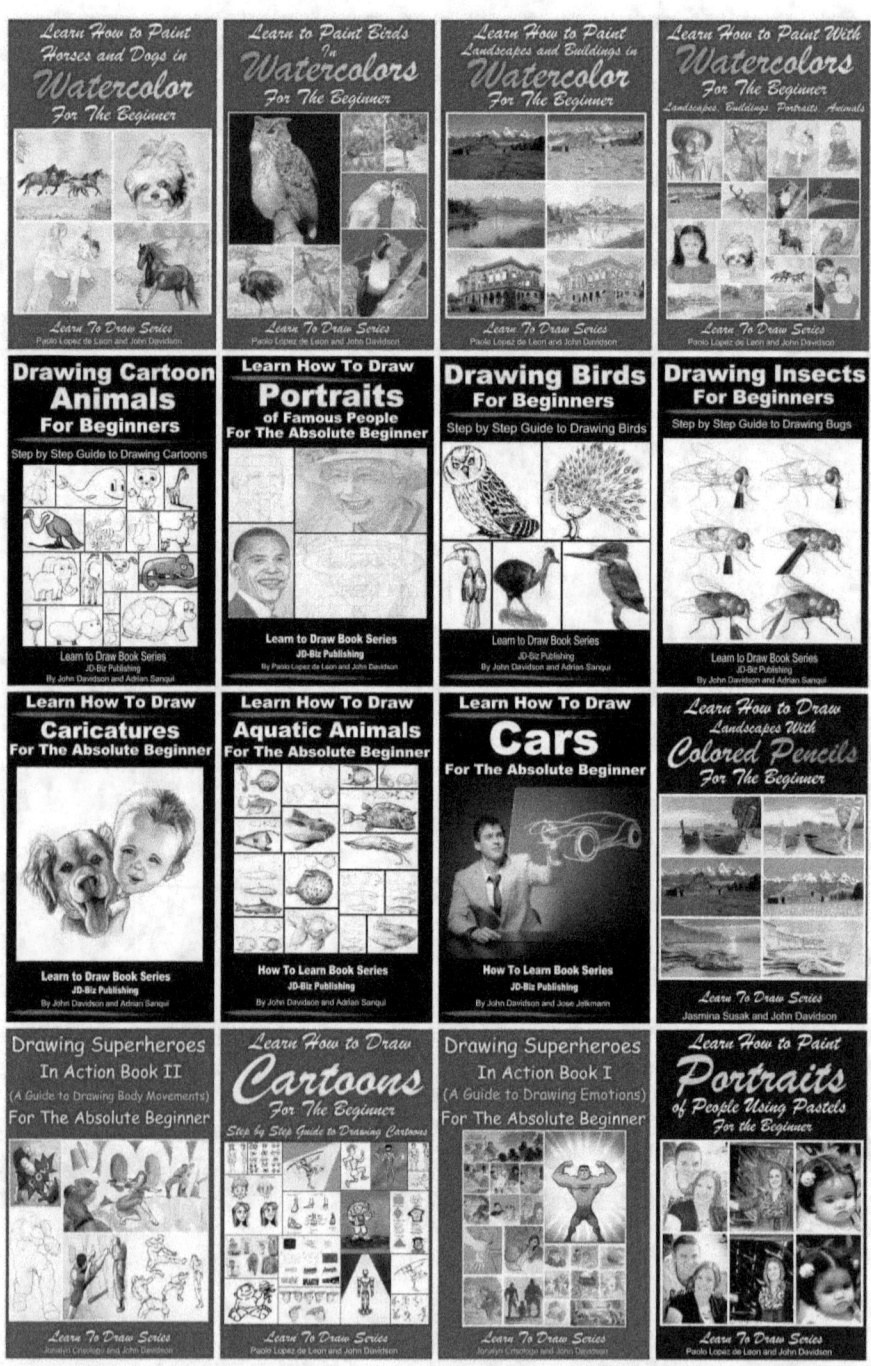

How to Build and Plan Books

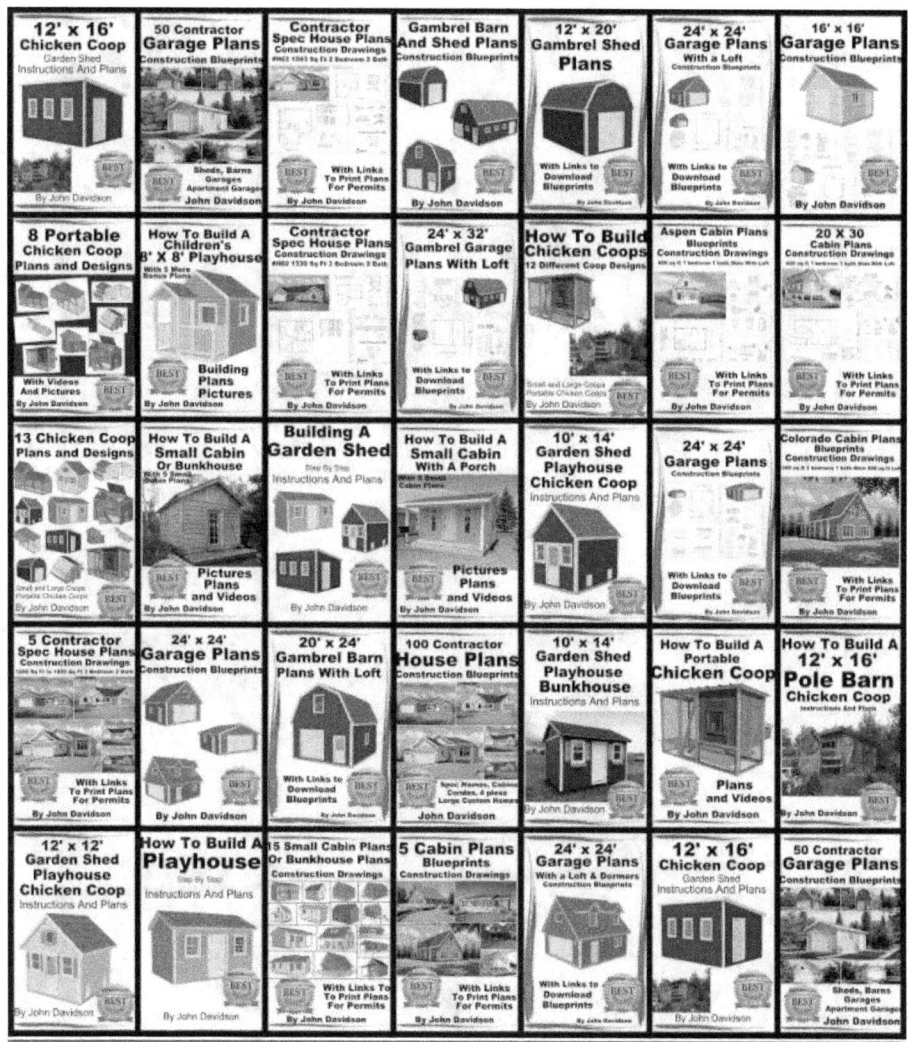

Entrepreneur Book Series

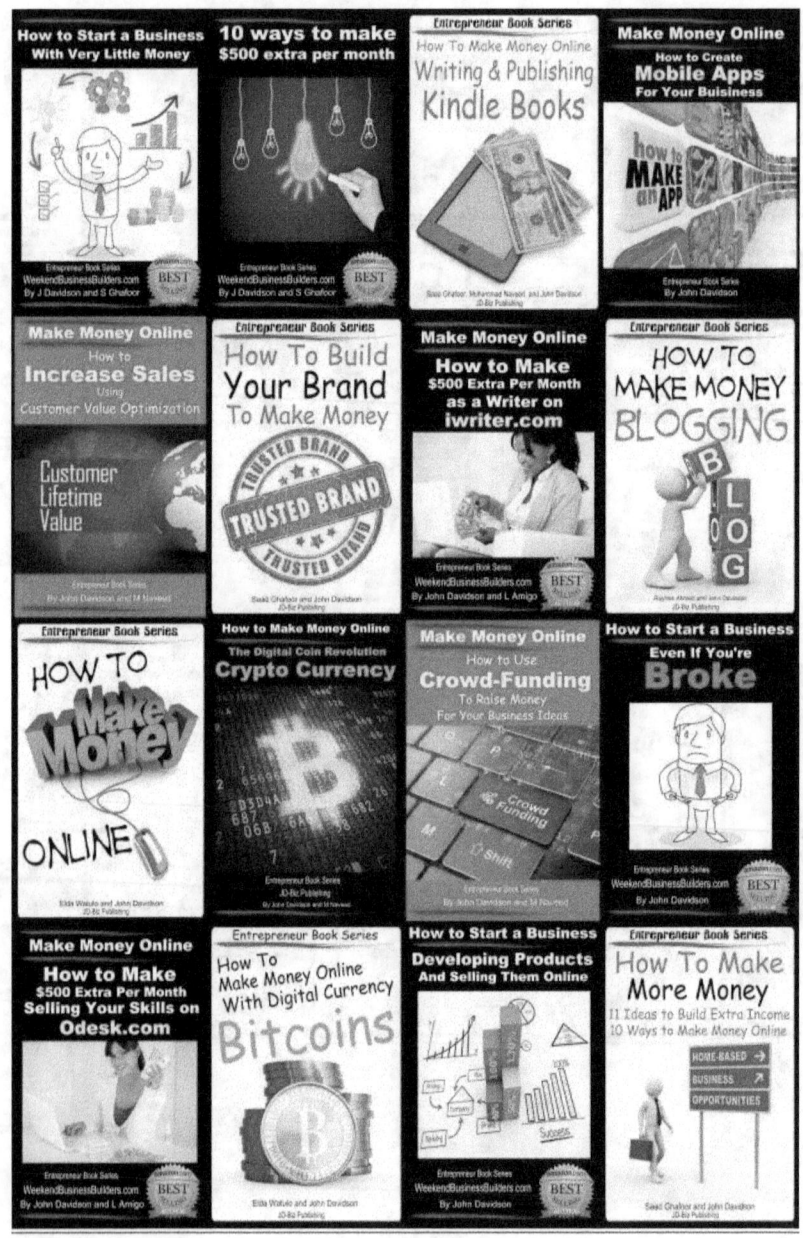

Publisher

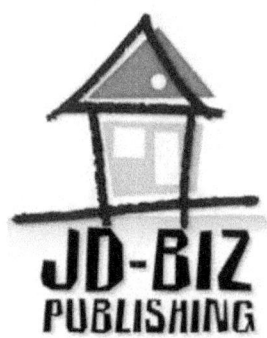

JD-Biz Corp

P O Box 374

Mendon, Utah 84325

http://www.jd-biz.com/

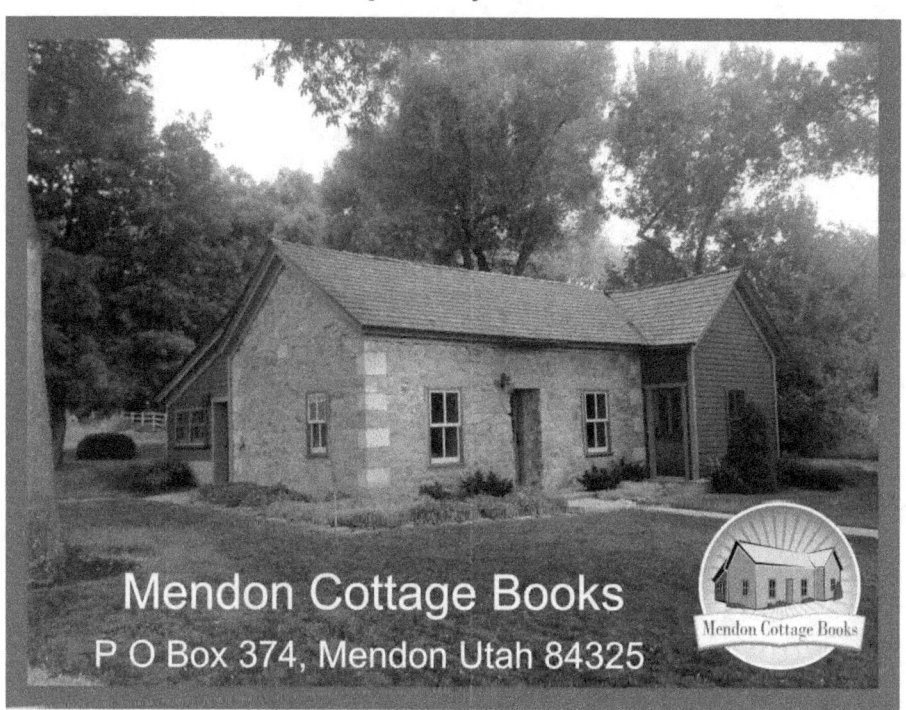

Mendon Cottage Books

P O Box 374, Mendon Utah 84325

www.ingramcontent.com/pod-product-compliance
Lightning Source LLC
Chambersburg PA
CBHW071138280526
45787CB00003B/1326